The Perimenopause Manual

Jacqui Sechiari

with
Benjamin Thomas

Table of Contents

Introduction	4
Why is this happening?	6
Why do we get these symptoms?	10
Why the Weight Gain?	14
What Are Our Biggest Health Issues in Menopause?	17
What can we do about it?	22
Who can help?	25
Hormone Replacement Therapy (HRT)	28
About the Author	32
References and Resources:	33

This is dedicated to all the women out there who thought they were getting Alzheimers, about to kill their kids, growing hairs on their chins, feeling like they had lost their identity, or just going mad. If you are searching for answers and found nothing that had all the helpful information in one place then this manual is for you.

This is just a starting point, and hopefully you'll be motivated into taking your journey further and to Rediscovering You.

Jacqui Sechiari

2020

Introduction

I'm Jacqui Sechiari, Health & Fitness and Certified Menopause Coach & author of your PM Manual.

In January 2020, I sent out a survey asking women (mainly in their 40's) how they felt about themselves currently and these are just some of the responses:

"Difficult to navigate and get the right information"

"I have never felt so alone"

"Frustrated, confused and old before my time - I'm 45"

"Feel like I have no joy or spark left in my life"

"Overwhelmed, unprepared and unsupported"

"Not living my best life right now and constantly trying to find the old me"

"It's just something we need to put up with, and it will be over eventually"

"It's all about adapting to a new reality. What once worked no longer works - it's not worse, or the end of the world, it's just different. I'm excited about the next stage of my life!"

I had 120 responses to this survey, and only 7 ladies responded with anything positive. This totally saddened and shocked me. The most common words or phrases that kept being repeated were,

"Confused, frustrated, overwhelmed"

"I don't know where to find any information"

"I Can't wait for it to be over"

"I want the old me back"

What it boils down to is:

- Knowing what you can and can't control

- Accepting that you cannot go back - and to start looking forwards!

- Realising that we don't have to '*put up with it!*' We should be informed, educated, supported and loving the journey into this new era

- Just like when we went through puberty, we will have to find a 'new normal,' and find a new you.

- Be excited, put yourself first, be informed and start taking care of you!

After reading these responses I felt compelled to put together this manual to end any confusion and give you the facts about *Why* this is happening, *Why* we get these symptoms, *What* we can do about it, *Who* can help and *Where* we can find like-minded women to talk to. So, here it is. Your own Perimenopause Manual. This is something I wish had been given to me as I was approaching 40, so I am writing this for all of you ladies who want to take control, rediscover you, and live your best lives!

- Jacqui x

Why is this happening?

Let's start with some of the symptoms that you may be experiencing. Look familiar?

- Anxiety
- Low Mood
- Depression
- Mood Swings
- Crying Spells
- Brain Fog
- Loss Of Confidence
- Irritability
- Loss Of Joy
- Poor Memory
- Poor Concentration
- Difficulty Sleeping
- Tired/no Energy
- Headaches
- Palpitations
- Hot Flushes
- Night Sweats

- Painful/Aching Joints
- Changes To Periods
- Vaginal Symptoms
- Urinary Symptoms
- Loss Of Libido
- Dry/itchy Skin
- Dry Eyes/ears
- Oral Health Changes
- Thinning Hair
- Weight Gain
- Feeling Dizzy/faint
- Tinnitus
- Restless Legs
- Change To Body Odour
- Increased Allergies
- Digestive Issues

Why is this happening?

Women are born with a finite amount of eggs. These eggs start to get released during puberty (and we all know about that, don't we?!). Puberty occurs when a part of the brain called the hypothalamus begins to produce a hormone (gonadotropin) that has an effect on the ovaries; causing an increase in oestrogen. When our periods start, this is a basic explanation of what happens during that monthly cycle:

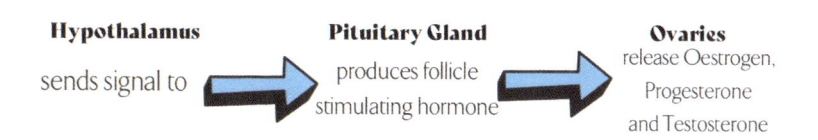

Hypothalamus sends signal to → **Pituitary Gland** produces follicle stimulating hormone → **Ovaries** release Oestrogen, Progesterone and Testosterone

As we get older, the egg reserve in our ovaries is depleting. The ovaries cannot work effectively due to ageing follicles and as a result, our sex hormones (oestrogen, progesterone and testosterone) start to decline. However, the body does not stop producing these hormones overnight and the process can even take several years- during which symptoms arise gradually. This gradual change is called the 'perimenopause'.

Perimenopause is a change in the levels of the hormones oestrogen, progesterone and testosterone.

This can start as early as 35 and continue until you have your final period. It is also the biggest opportunity for personal growth and empowerment since puberty!

The menopause refers to that time in every woman's life when her periods have stopped (no period for 12 months) and her ovaries lose their reproductive function. Usually, this occurs between the ages of 45 and 55. In the UK the average age is 51.

In a few exceptional cases women may become menopausal in their 30s, or even younger. This is then known as a premature menopause, or premature ovarian insufficiency.

Some women may have had a hysterectomy and, at the same time, surgical removal of the ovaries for various medical reasons. Removal of the ovaries will create an immediate menopause, whatever the patient's age, and all the symptoms and risks associated with a natural menopause will apply to these women. (1)

Peri Menopause
Usually occurs in your 40's
Can last 6 years or more!
Oestrogen levels dip irregularly
Periods become unpredictable and less frequent
Ends 1 year after your final period

Menopause
Officially (and medically) when you are period free for 12 straight months
Average age for Menopause in the UK is 51
Oestrogen levels drop markedly, naturally causing certain changes in the body

Post Menopause
Any time after Menopause is considered post menopause
Oestrogen levels continue to drop, causing symptoms such as hot flushes and bone loss

Diagnosing the (Peri) Menopause

These rules relate to the UK only (according to NICE- National Institute for Health and Care Excellence- guidelines)

It's not always easy to confirm that you are in perimenopause or that menopause has actually happened, especially if you are using the contraceptive pill, Mirena coil or anything that affects your hormone levels. If you are not using anything that alters your hormones, you will be considered to be "in menopause" once you have been period free for 12 months. Technically, menopause only lasts for one day as anything after this point is considered post menopause.

Most doctors will evaluate a woman's menopausal status according to her symptoms, pattern of periods, and medical records. It is possible to take a blood test to measure levels of a hormone known as FSH (follicle-stimulating hormone). This hormone is released from the pituitary gland and stimulates the growth of eggs in the ovaries. FSH causes oestrogen and progesterone to be produced. As our egg follicles age and become depleted, the signal between the pituitary gland and ovaries becomes weaker, causing FSH to become elevated. However, while elevated FSH levels may be a sign of the menopause, the test is not always accurate, especially during perimenopause when hormone levels fluctuate daily and results can't be guaranteed so measurement of FSH is not required to diagnose perimenopause or menopause in women aged over 45 years. (2)

Why do we get these symptoms?

For most of us, menopause is a natural life stage that we all go through. Every woman's experience is unique and personal to them. Some will suffer from all of the symptoms and some just a few. So why do we suffer from these symptoms?

Let's take a look at the major hormones that are at play and what they are responsible for:

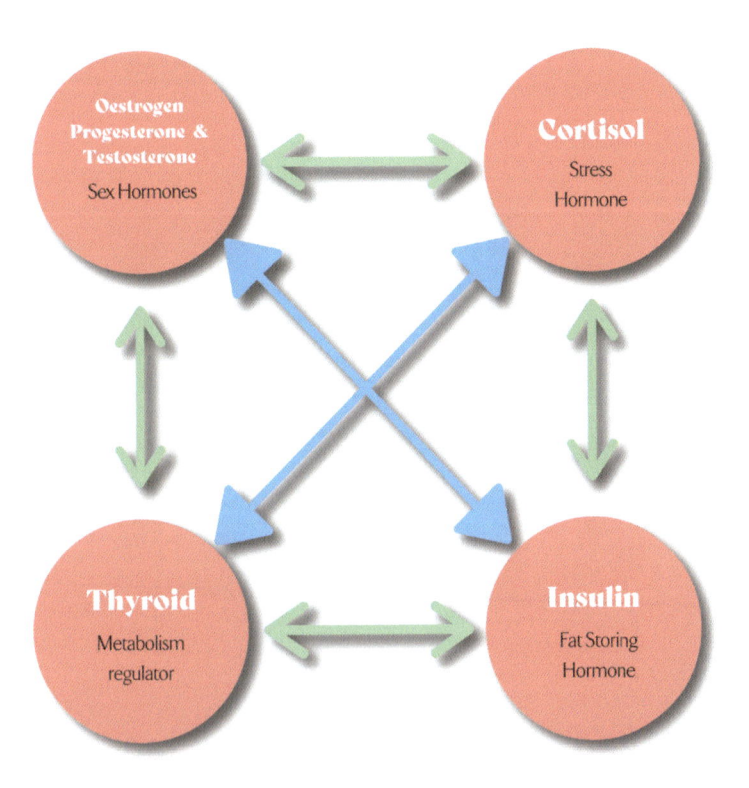

Oestrogen Progesterone & Testosterone — Sex Hormones

Cortisol — Stress Hormone

Thyroid — Metabolism regulator

Insulin — Fat Storing Hormone

Let's start with the sex hormones, Oestrogen, Progesterone and Testosterone. The main player here is of course, Oestrogen, (think of her as the 'party animal') which has over 400 different functions in the body. In women, almost every cell in the body has Oestrogen receptors, but they are more concentrated in the brain, heart, liver, skin, bones, breasts and reproductive systems.

It stimulates the growth of an egg follicle and helps to lubricate the vagina. It helps to maintain the body's temperature, regulate the part of the brain linked to sexual development and enhance the effect of the brain's 'feel good' chemicals. It improves the thickness and quality of the skin (and hair!) as well as the collagen content which prevents ageing. It helps to protect bone/connective tissue strength and prevent bone loss. It regulates cholesterol production in the liver, helping to protect the heart and arteries.

Progesterone is the more 'calming' hormone that we get lots of when we are pregnant, it is an anti-anxiety hormone which protects the lining of the womb and helps to relax our soft tissues and smooth muscles.

Then we have Testosterone (yes ladies, it's not just for men!) which helps with our libido, energy levels and is important for muscle and bone strength.

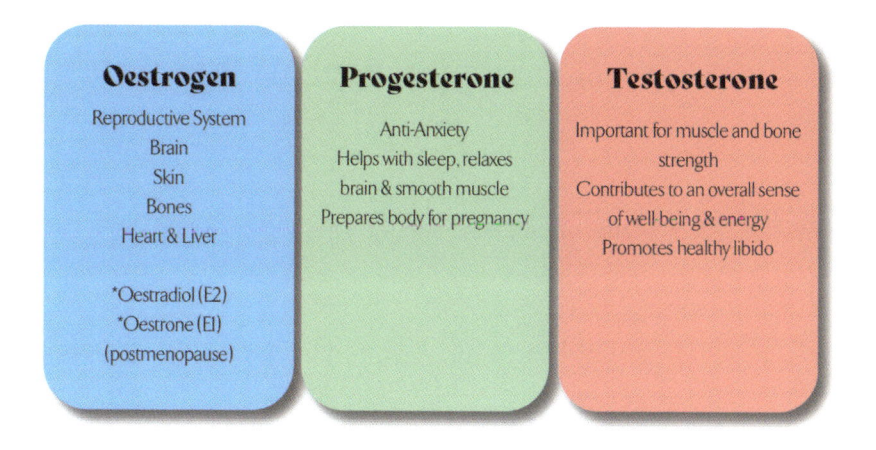

Oestrogen	Progesterone	Testosterone
Reproductive System	Anti-Anxiety	Important for muscle and bone strength
Brain	Helps with sleep, relaxes brain & smooth muscle	Contributes to an overall sense of well-being & energy
Skin	Prepares body for pregnancy	Promotes healthy libido
Bones		
Heart & Liver		
*Oestradiol (E2)		
*Oestrone (E1)		
(postmenopause)		

Are you starting to see why we may be having some of those symptoms outlined above?? BUT it isn't just the sex hormones that we need to consider.....

The thyroid (which produces thyroxine) regulates our body temperature and is critical for metabolism. Hypothyroidism (an underactive thyroid) is a condition that affects the thyroid gland and people with this condition produce a low amount of thyroid hormone. Hypothyroidism and menopause share some symptoms so it is important that you 'test- don't guess' if you are having symptoms such as: thinning of head hair, depression, dry skin, forgetfulness, weight gain, muscle/joint aches and pains, fatigue. Declining oestrogen levels can affect thyroid function. In a peer reviewed study from 2011, researchers found that oestrogen levels might affect thyroid function and lead to thyroid disorders due to the role that oestrogen levels have on thyroid receptors.

Insulin is released by the pancreas and controls your blood sugar levels. Insulin is released after eating to escort the sugar out of the blood and into the muscle cells to be burned for energy. It is also your fat storing hormone. As you lose oestrogen, you become more insulin resistant, (3) so your body pumps out more insulin, which in turn triggers more fat storage.

Cortisol is released from the adrenal glands and is our stress or 'fight or flight' hormone to prepare the body for an emergency. It tells the liver to quickly dump a lot of sugar into the bloodstream to be used for energy and all other hormones are temporarily 'ignored' until the emergency is dealt with. This is a BIG deal because the brain can't distinguish between 'real' danger and every day stresses. Elevated cortisol levels result in:

1) Increase blood sugar levels to keep energy going therefore increased insulin resistance (this can lead to diabetes)
2) Increased cravings and appetite and increased inflammation.
3) Reduced production of thyroid stimulating hormone and sex hormones
4) Digestion stops working properly

Cortisol	**Insulin**	**Thyroid**
Stress Hormone	Controls blood sugar	Controls metabolism and body temperature
Converts protein into glucose to boost blood sugar levels	Releases insulin from pancreas and takes sugar to muscles, liver and fat	Produces T4 (Thyroxin)
Other hormones temporarily ignored	Fat storing hormone	Body converts this to T3, primarily in liver and gut. This is the 'active' form the body can use
Suppresses immune, digestive and reproductive systems		

So, hopefully we can see that menopause isn't just about your ovaries – it's about ageing, your stress, your health over your lifetime and how ALL hormones work together to help you survive!

The most powerful connection is between your thyroid, pituitary and adrenal hormones! (the HPA axis). You need to learn how to rebalance all of the hormones that are produced on this axis.

So, if menopause is a natural life stage that we all go through, why do we suffer from these symptoms and health changes?

Let's just say that modern day life doesn't help. Most women who are around 45 now have been juggling a life of career, pregnancy, kids, partner, cooking, exercise, house renovating, travelling, partying, ageing parents (or deaths), managing finances....the list goes on. Up to this point we don't really notice any issues. But when one hormone gets out balance, the sh*t hits the fan because they are all connected. And that's when the fun begins!

The life that we have lived contributes to our symptoms. That includes all the emotional, physical and nutritional choices that we have made will have contributed to our symptoms. Look at what 'our generation' have been exposed to: sugar, low fat products, convenience foods, modern medicine and antibiotics, alcohol, smoking, using the contraceptive pill, stress, told to eat less and exercise more. Our lifestyle over decades has increased inflammation on the body and so does ageing. The result for many women is that this past lifestyle and declining oestrogen has a dramatic effect on the brain, heart, gut, liver muscle and joint health in mid-life.

Why the Weight Gain?

Many women start to gain weight during their 40's despite eating and exercising the same as they always have. It also tends to be stored around the middle, giving an 'apple' shape to the body rather than the 'hourglass' shape we may have been used to. What is the natural reaction to this? To eat less calories and exercise more? - but it doesn't work. We need to understand what other factors are playing a role in this weight gain.

Metabolism

Muscle mass typically diminishes with age, while fat increases. Losing muscle mass slows the rate at which your body uses calories (metabolism). This can make it more challenging to maintain a healthy weight. If you continue to eat as you always have and don't increase your muscle mass, you're likely to gain weight. Added to that, as oestrogen drops this has an effect on the rate of protein synthesis meaning it becomes more difficult for your body to synthesise the protein you eat into the muscle that you need.

Insulin Sensitivity

Oestrogen and progesterone have an impact on some of the fat burning and fat storing hormones. Oestrogen makes the body more insulin sensitive so as oestrogen declines women become more insulin resistant (3); your body pumps out more insulin, which in turn triggers more fat storage. This puts you on the blood-sugar rollercoaster of surges and drops that can leave you fatigued and hungry all the time.

Cravings

For those of you who have been pregnant or got weird cravings during your periods, guess what? It's related to hormones! In the brain we have gaba (neuro relaxing transmitter), dopamine (focussing brain chemical) and serotonin (self-esteem and relaxing chemical) which all fall during your period and during perimenopause. There are oestrogen receptors all over the brain and so this decline can cause mood changes and cravings which make it even more difficult for women at (peri) menopause to stay on the same diet and for it to work the way it once did.

Stress – Increased Cortisol

Oestrogen and progesterone together make women less responsive to cortisol (our stress hormone). Prolonged raised cortisol makes us increase fat storage around the middle. When we are stressed (emotional, or physical), our body goes into survival mode as it thinks you are in danger (it doesn't know the difference between ACTUAL danger and emotional stress). All other hormones are inhibited as the body is in survival mode, therefore oestrogen and progesterone decline further which just spirals the situation further.

Sleep Disturbances

Progesterone has direct sedative effects and is declining rapidly. Oestrogen increases REM sleep, decreases the number of times you wake in the night and helps to regulate your body temperature. As these hormones decline, sleep is compromised. Lack of quality sleep triggers a cortisol spike, decreases insulin sensitivity and has adverse effects on overall well-being. Focusing on good sleep hygiene is paramount for weight loss.

Fat Cells Make Oestrogen

As the body starts to produce less and less oestrogen in the ovaries, oestrogen is produced in other areas of the body, namely the adrenal glands and fat tissue. As oestrogen levels drop, body fat is redistributed from the hips, thighs, and buttocks (where it used to be stored as a fuel reserve for breastfeeding) to the abdomen. Excessive amounts of visceral fat increase inflammation in the body and ultimately contribute to several conditions, including heart disease, diabetes, and cancer.

What Are Our Biggest Health Issues in Menopause?

Brain Changes in Menopause

Menopause symptoms are neurological - part of the neuroendocrine system. The ovaries and brain talk to each other. As our eggs decline, production of oestrogen declines. Oestrogen is key for bringing energy to the brain. Oestrogen helps to stimulate the production and transportation of serotonin around the body, and prevents its break down. Therefore, when oestrogen levels are low serotonin is low and an unstable mood and anxiety can develop. The ageing process also means that our memory is affected.

What can we do to help our brain?

Eat the right foods. Foods high in Tryptophan can help to make serotonin. Physical exercise produces that 'high' feeling. Exercise affects the brain in many ways. It increases heart rate, which pumps more oxygen to the brain. It aids the release of hormones which provide an excellent environment for the growth of brain cells. Exercise also promotes brain plasticity by stimulating growth of new connections between cells in many important cortical areas of the brain. Learn to stimulate the brain with word games or learning something new. All it takes is 15 minutes a day.

Heart Changes in Menopause

Cardiovascular disease is very common in women. It is still under diagnosed and under treated. Many women are not having their risk factors for cardiovascular disease properly addressed. The risk of cardiovascular disease greatly increases after the menopause when

The Role of Oestrogen

Helps to regulate cholesterol
Protects lining of artery walls
Reduces risk of plaque build-up inside arteries

Declining Oestrogen Causes

Increase in LDL (bad) cholesterol
Increased risk of arteries narrowing
Increase in Blood Pressure

oestrogen levels reduce. (3,4)

During and after the menopause, a woman's body gradually produces less oestrogen than it used to. This increases the risk of the coronary arteries narrowing whereas it previously protected the lining of the artery walls reducing the build-up of plaque. This increases your risk of developing coronary heart disease, or a circulatory condition such as stroke and increases your blood pressure. (5)

What can we do to help our heart?

It is a muscle. It needs to work out. Try and get breathless for 10 minutes a day. It doesn't matter what you do.

British Heart Foundation funded research, at Oxford University, showed middle-aged women could significantly lower their risk of heart disease and stroke by exercising even just two or three times a week. The study, of over one million UK women, showed women who did strenuous physical activity two to three times a week, or any activity up to four to six times a week, had around a 20% lower risk of coronary heart disease, stroke and blood clots compared to women who were inactive

Bone Changes in Menopause

According to the International Osteoporosis Foundation, in the UK one in two women over the age of 50 will experience osteoporotic fractures. (6) That's 50%!! Low bone mass is usually caused by a combination of factors, typically including older age, nutrient deficiencies, physical inactivity, high levels of stress, existing health conditions and others.

Bone Health Facts

Peak bone mass achieved by age of 25
1 in 2 women over 50 will experience osteoporotic fractures!

Contributing Factors

Age
Gender
Race
Family History
Medications
Physical Activity
Smoking
Alcohol Intake

Bone is living tissue that has to be constantly repaired and renewed because of microscopic damage that occurs with daily physical activity. This process of renewal is called bone turnover and is carried out by two sets of cells; one set (osteoclasts) breaks down bone tissue whilst the other set (osteoblasts) lay down new bone. The two processes are linked together so that they balance each other. If there is a relative increase in bone removal, as happens following menopause, then bone tissue is lost and bones become thinner. There is gradual loss of bone with ageing in adults, but major bone loss in women occurs with loss of oestrogen at the menopause. (7)

What can we do to help our bones?

Get a decent nights sleep, around 7-8 hours of uninterrupted sleep a night. Sleep is when the healing and magic happens. Get enough Vitamin D as this promotes calcium absorption in the gut. It is also needed for bone growth and bone remodelling by osteoblasts and osteoclasts. Weight bearing exercises are ESSENTIAL for both health bones and to improve muscle mass as we age. Just start with bodyweight exercises and progress from there. All it takes is 5 minutes a day!

If there is a family history of osteopenia or osteoporosis or you have concerns because of previous medications etc, diagnosis can be made before a fracture has occurred using a DEXA scan. You would need to speak to your GP about this.

Liver Changes in Menopause

The volume and blood flow of the liver gradually decrease with ageing. According to studies using ultrasound, the liver volume decreases by 20–40% as one gets older. Such changes are related to a decline in the blood flow in the liver, in that those aged 65 years or higher showed an approximately 35% decrease in the blood volume of the liver compared with those aged less than 40 years (8). There is an interplay of hormonal issues and ageing that create a unique path for development of liver disease in menopausal women. Before menopause, oestradiol is the predominant and most potent form of oestrogen. Post menopause, however, oestrone, a much weaker form of oestrogen, predominates and is produced via fat cells and in the liver. In menopause, the interplay of reductions in oestrogen levels along with biochemical effects of the ageing process foster an environment that increases the propensity for damage within the liver. (9)

It is the role of the liver to remove toxins, help to update many of the B vitamins, regulate our hormones and metabolism, fight infections and diseases and remove old oestrogen. If the liver can't get rid of the cholesterol, toxins and oestrogen it gets stored in the fat cells. Women have more fat cells around the abdominal region. The fat gets taken to the visceral fat around the organs which can lead to other health issues such as heart disease, diabetes, cancer and high blood pressure.

What can we do to help our liver?

Treat it with respect! It has a lot of work to do. Reduce toxins such as alcohol, certain medications, cleaning and skin products. Eat plenty of cruciferous vegetables and green leafy veg, good fats such as oily fish, olive oil, walnuts, avocados and non refined carbohydrates.

What can we do about it?

First of all – DON'T LOOK BACK – you can't go that way. You need to look to the future. You need to focus on what you need now at this time of life. You need to change. You need to change your beliefs. You need to find your purpose. Consistency is key. Forming life changing habits is key. Here are the key areas to focus on:

Reducing Sources of Stress (emotional & physical)

- Radical self-care – start putting yourself first
- Learn some diaphragmatic, deep breathing techniques as these really help with stress and stimulate your parasympathetic nervous system
- Bring some joy and laughter into your life
- Learn how to meditate or some mindfulness techniques, just 5 or 10 minutes per day.
- Stop dieting and pounding your body with too much exercise. These are physical stressors on the body.

Prioritising Sleep Quality

- The long-term effects of sleep deprivation are real. It drains your mental abilities and puts your physical health at real risk. Science has linked poor slumber with all kinds of health problems, from weight gain to a weakened immune system.(10)

- Get into a healthy sleep habit NOW! Eliminate blue lights from the bedroom, darken the room, go to bed and get up at the same time every day (where possible), relax before bedtime.

Movement for muscles, bones, heart and balance

- Focus on joint health, especially around the common fracture sites (wrist, pelvis)
- Strength matters for healthy muscles, bones and metabolism
- Walking is great for this stage in life as it gets you outside and helps with insulin resistance.
- Aerobic exercise matters. Get breathless for at least 10 mins per day to protect the heart
- Flexibility and balance matter. Yoga is great for the body and the mind.
- Pelvic health matters. No-one wants to wear Tena Pads!

Below is a summary of the best exercises for muscle and bone strengthening and balance

Which types of Physical Activities are effective in developing muscle and bone strength and balance?

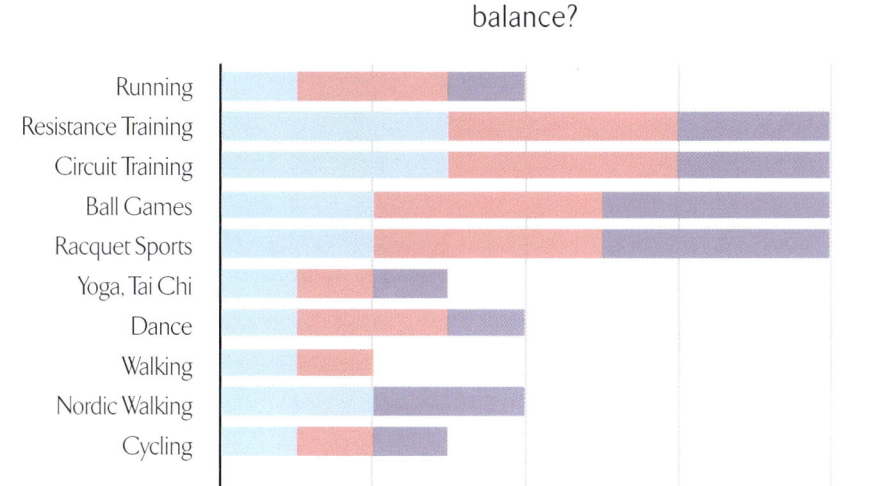

- Running
- Resistance Training
- Circuit Training
- Ball Games
- Racquet Sports
- Yoga, Tai Chi
- Dance
- Walking
- Nordic Walking
- Cycling

Improvement in Muscle Function   Improvement in Bone Health
Improvement in Balance

Source: Public Health England & Centre for Ageing Better

Reduce Inflammation and Toxicity

- Go organic where you can, as toxins mess with your hormones
- Use natural products on the skin, as the skin absorbs creams and lotions
- Use natural cleaning products in the house
- Ditch the plastic!
- Try to quit (or reduce) smoking and reduce your alcohol intake

Change your diet, stop dieting

- Get off the sugar-stress rollercoaster
- Do not go on a low-fat diet! Good, healthy fats are ESSENTIAL at this time of life for hormone production. Think extra virgin olive oils, flax oil, avocados, nuts and seeds,
- Eat meals that contain all food groups at EVERY meal (protein, fibre, fats) and adopt more of a Mediterranean Diet (no, not pizza & pasta!)Make gut health a priority to lower inflammation
- Eat foods containing phytoestrogens (natural oestrogen) like linseed, sesame seeds, soy products (best kinds are organic, fermented products like miso and Tamari)
- Cut out processed foods and refined carbohydrates. Focus on wholemeal, seeded, natural carbohydrates and legumes – brown/wild rice, chick peas, lentils, beans, peas, quinoa

Social Connection Matters

- Women need other women! Find your tribe, a support group of likeminded women so that you can share experiences and support each other
- Anxiety can be one of the worst symptoms for some women who stop going out and seeing anyone. Reach out locally or online and ask for help

Who can help?

Ladies, the above options are, of course, changes in lifestyle factors that can help to ease your symptoms of menopause. We can't continue to try and live like a 20 or 30-year-old and expect to feel good. We should eat and exercise for our changing, ageing bodies and hormones. I firmly believe that every woman should strive to be in their prime health at this stage of life and not settle for anything less. PUT YOUR HEALTH FIRST!

I also believe that you need to take OWNERSHIP of your own health. I can tell you, and tell you, and tell you again what to do. But YOU are one that has to DO it. You have to change your habits and it won't happen overnight so be patient with yourselves. Be kind to yourselves. Invest in yourselves.

I offer lifestyle change programmes for women which help you to take back control and rediscover you again. They provide a foundation for you, to focus on creating daily habits based on your current symptoms, then provide you with an ongoing plan for growth and change.

These are delivered via an app and are focused on making small daily changes whilst being supported by me and other women who are part of our Rediscover You Community. Continued support is offered via a closed Facebook group which keeps you up to date with the latest research and resources. You can find more information and sign up to the newsletter via my website: jacquisechiari.com

If you have any underlying health conditions or have more complex issues, I would recommend finding a good nutritional therapist that specialises in hormones. In the past I have used Catherine Pohl who can offer consultations virtually (I am not getting ANY commission out of this. I only recommend people I have used personally), but obviously feel free to find anyone who you feel comfortable with.

Your doctor should be able to help and offer advice. However, not all are up to date with the latest guidance on diagnosis and treatment.

The following information is for the UK only. International equivalents may vary.

I always recommend asking if they are up date with the latest NICE guidelines or if you can see a GP who has a special interest in women's health. Please do your research before going to your GP so that you are aware of what the guidelines say and be prepared. Do NOT let them fob you off with anti-depressants.

Here (menopausesupport.co.uk/?p=1668) are some great guidelines on how to prepare for your GP appointment.

There are Menopause Specialists that you can see for free on the NHS but there is usually a long waiting so get your name down now if this is something you would like to do. You can check where your nearest Menopause Specialist is located here (https://thebms.org.uk/find-a-menopause-specialist/)

There are also Private Menopause Specialists that can help you for a fee. Due to the current situation with COVID 19, many of these are offering virtual appointments. If you decide to go down this route and you are given a prescription for HRT, you should be able to get future prescriptions through the NHS (depending on what is prescribed). I have had the pleasure of working with Dr Naomi Potter, a GP and private Menopause Specialist, who can offer virtual consultations.

Where can we meet likeminded women?

There are lots of Facebook groups or forums that you can join.

Dr Naomi Potter, GP and Menopause Specialist, has a free forum that you can join here (https://www.drnaomipotter.com/menopauseforum).

Menopause Matters also has a free forum and a magazine that you can subscribe to. There are loads of other great resources on here too.

Diane Danzebrink has an excellent website called My Menopause Support and a Facebook Group (Menopause Support Network) that you can join and also has a podcast which is well worth a listen.

Louise Newson (The Menopause Doctor) has an excellent website with fantastic resources and information especially if you have an appointment with a GP! She also has a great podcast which covers lots of different and helpful topics.

The British Menopause Society (BMS) have a patient arm called Women's Health Concern
and their website is full of resources, videos, help and advice and events that you could attend. (the American equivalent of this is The North American Menopause Society NAMS)

For women who are suffering from premature menopause (earlier than the age of 40), also known as premature ovarian failure and/or premature ovarian insufficiency (POI), there is a charity called The Daisy Network who have an excellent website and support network.

Menopause Café (www.menopausecafe.net)was set up for ANYONE to meet up and discuss all things menopause over a cup of coffee or tea and a piece of cake. They are also running Online menopause cafes.

Hormone Replacement Therapy (HRT)

Learning how to change your lifestyle at this crucial stage of life is important to prime you and keep you as healthy as possible for the rest of your life whether or not you decide to take HRT. You will probably find that with a few tweaks and habit changes, many of your symptoms will ease or disappear, as they may be due to stress, lack of sleep, weight gain, sedentary lifestyle, the wrong diet and not necessarily down to lack of oestrogen.

However, if your symptoms are so debilitating that you need medical help, then you should seek it. Please make sure that you are educated and armed with the correct information concerning HRT before you visit your GP. Here is some basic information regarding HRT that is available in the UK now.

What is HRT?

Hormone Replacement Therapy is to replace the sex hormones (oestrogen, progesterone & testosterone) that are declining. Women are now living longer then ever before. The average age of death of women in the UK is around 82 so we are likely to live around 30 years after menopause. As discussed already, these hormones (especially oestrogen) have an important role in the blood vessels, bones, brain, skin, hair and many more.

What hormones are there in HRT?

The most important hormone is oestrogen which is mainly produced by the ovaries until the eggs are depleted. All types of HRT should contain some oestrogen. If you see a GP that isn't offering you oestrogen you need to question why. (for example, you may be offered the progesterone only pill or Merina coil which only contains progesterone.)

In the past, oestrogen used to be derived from pregnant horses' urine and was prescribed as a tablet. The oestrogen that is offered now is usually prescribed as a patch, gel or spray so it is absorbed through the skin and it is Body Identical. This means it is the same structure as the hormones we produce ourselves and is made from yams which is a natural product.

Oestrogen on its own can lead to thickening of the lining of the womb (which can lead to some cancers) so if a woman still has their womb (not had a hysterectomy) they also have to take a type of progesterone to protect the lining of womb. With progesterone, there are different types.

- Progestogens. These are 'synthetic' progesterone (not the same structure as we produce)
- Progesterone. These are the body identical type (same structure as we produce)

Testosterone is also produced by ovaries and this gradually declines as we get older and with menopause. Some women also benefit from having testosterone replacement too.

Why is there so much controversy around HRT?

In the past women were prescribed HRT relatively freely and this was the older type of HRT (horses' urine and synthetic progestogen). Worldwide lots of women were feeling the benefits and feeling better and their longer-term heath seemed to benefit (better heart health, bones and brain health). In response, the US conducted a multimillion-dollar study in 2002 (WHI -Women's Health Initiative Study) to see if older women would benefit from taking HRT as they knew that younger women were benefitting already. The average age of the women was 63, which is 12 years older than the average natural menopause age, many of them were overweight and obese and many of them had had heart disease before the study. They were already high risk because of their history and weight. The study looked at 'placebo' compared to HRT. The HRT given was a tablet oestrogen derived from horse's urine and a synthetic progestogen (they were combined as a pill). Some women in the study had had a hysterectomy and weren't given the progestogen as they don't need it. The doses that were given were higher doses than would be prescribed now. What they found in the study was that some of these women were experiencing heart attacks and there was a small increase in the risk of breast cancer. The study was stopped very abruptly and it was leaked to the press before any good researcher could look at it to analyse the study properly. The headlines stated that taking HRT causes heart attacks and breast cancer and women very quickly stopped taking it.

Subsequently the study was looked at properly at what they found was that:

- The younger women who took HRT within 10 years of their menopause had a far lower risk of heart disease, dementia and osteoporosis,
- The women who only took oestrogen had a lower risk of breast cancer
- The women who started HRT after 10 years of menopause had a small increased risk of having a heart attack, especially those who took the combined pill (oestrogen & progestogen). There was also small increased risk of breast cancer in this group of women.

Fast forward 18 years, during which this study and others have been analysed over and over, the overall conclusion is: (12)

- Women wishing to start HRT should carefully discuss the benefits and risks of treatment with their doctor to see what is right for them, taking into account their age, medical history, risk factors and personal preferences.
- For the majority of women who use HRT for the short-term treatment of symptoms of the menopause, the benefits of treatment are considered to outweigh the risks.
- The lowest effective HRT dose should be taken, with duration of use depending on the clinical reasons for use.
- HRT remains licensed for osteoporosis prevention and can be considered the treatment of choice for women starting treatment below age 60 years, and especially for those with a premature menopause.
- Women on HRT should be re-assessed by their doctor at least annually. For some women, long-term use of HRT may be necessary for continued symptom relief and quality of life.

Understanding the Risks of Breast cancer

There are other risk factors for breast cancer such as being overweight, drinking alcohol, being inactive, taking the contraceptive pill, family history, exposure to radiation. This is why it's super important to stay a healthy weight, exercise and reduce alcohol. Here is a very informative chart which shows the risks of taking HRT compared to other lifestyle factors.

Synthetic vs Body Identical

When women take a synthetic progestogen, they have risks associated with them. These synthetic progestogens when given with oestrogen have a very small increased risk of clots, heart disease, raising cholesterol levels, breast cancer. So, is there an alternative?

Micronized progesterone (Utrogestan in the UK) is body identical progesterone. Micronized means the particle sizes are made very small which increases the surface area of the drug and that means it more easily absorbed in the body. They are taken as capsules. Studies have shown that the natural progesterone doesn't have an increased risk of clots, heart disease and for the first 5 years of taking them no increased risk of breast cancer. After 5 years, there is a small increased risk but not as high as with the older type of HRT.

There are lots of different ways of taking it and lots of different brands, so you need to discuss this with your GP and find the right one works for YOU. (Please do not confuse BODY identical with BIO Identical HRT which is NOT regulated in the UK and extremely expensive). You can read more about the different types of HRT here

Ladies, I hope this has been useful for you. Thank you for your time. Now go and have the BEST "REST OF YOUR LIFE" and remember, "small changes, big difference".

Jacqui x

About the Author

I'm Jacqui Sechiari, Health & Fitness and Certified Menopause Coach and author of your PM Manual.

I was 41 when I had my second child after suffering from 5 miscarriages after my first. I'd kind of given up hope and was on my 'last chance'. I think mentally I just couldn't take anymore. I never had a problem getting pregnant, but since my first pregnancy I had never managed to get past 12 weeks. I'd reached the stage of almost giving up. I prayed. I got pregnant. I prayed again. I got past 12 weeks. Then I reached 20 weeks. I still believe to this day that it was divine intervention, but that's another story.

Age 43 I realised that my body felt different than after my first baby. I blamed post baby hormones. By now I had retrained into the health and fitness industry and gained my personal training qualification. We didn't learn about hormones specific to females. We didn't learn about symptoms like mood swings, brain fog, irritability, forgetfulness, trouble sleeping, water retention, PMS, weight gain, loss of libido, decreased sense of wellbeing, depression, headaches.

I started doing my own research and fell into the 'perimenopause' world. I was shocked. Like standing there open mouthed shocked...... WHY DID I NOT KNOW ABOUT THIS? I remember at school we were separated from the boys and taken off into a room where we talked about periods and tampons and sanitary towels and given a little leaflet to take away and read. Why isn't there a little manual given to us all at a certain age to explain what happens when our periods end and not just begin? Why are there ante natal classes for giving birth but nothing for perimenopause to prepare you? I mean, it's LIFE CHANGING right?

I hope this manual has inspired and empowered you to start making small changes in your lives now so you can thrive for the rest of it. We are all unique individuals, each on our journey and you need to focus on what is right for YOU right now. Remember to start small and focus on your biggest concerns first. Small changes, big difference!

References and Resources:

Instagram:

@jacquisechiarimenopause

Website:

jacquisechiari.com

Email:

contact@jacquisechiari.com

Facebook:

facebook.com/rediscoveryoumenopause

1. https://www.womens-health-concern.org/help-and-advice/factsheets/menopause/
2. Nice Guidelines Diagnosis
3. https://www.ncbi.nlm.nih.gov/pmc/articles/PMC2810543/
4. https://www.bhf.org.uk/informationsupport/support/women-with-a-heart-condition/menopause-and-heart-disease
5. https://pubmed.ncbi.nlm.nih.gov/29338561/
6. https://www.iofbonehealth.org/facts-statistics#category-22
7. https://theros.org.uk/information-and-support/understanding-osteoporosis/causes-of-osteoporosis-and-broken-bones/

8. https://www.ncbi.nlm.nih.gov/pmc/articles/PMC4736713/
9. https://www.ncbi.nlm.nih.gov/pmc/articles/PMC4491951/
10. https://www.healthline.com/health/sleep-deprivation/effects-on-body
11. https://assets.publishing.service.gov.uk/government/uploads/system/uploads/attachment_data/file/721874/MBSBA_evidence_review.pdf
12. https://www.womens-health-concern.org/help-and-advice/factsheets/hrt-know-benefits-risks/

Designed and Edited by Benjamin Thomas of [Jambon Beurre](#)

Editors Note: As a 24 year old guy it was a pleasure working with Jacqui but I think I now know more about menopause than any other guy my age on the planet. Enjoy!

Printed in Great Britain
by Amazon